IBS Management Blueprint

A Holistic Approach to Understanding, Managing, and Thriving with Irritable Bowel Syndrome

Ivana Decker

Table of Contents

INTRODUCTION

In my years of practice as a gastroenterologist, I've been privileged to share in the deeply personal journeys of countless individuals navigating the challenges of Irritable Bowel Syndrome (IBS). This experience has not only deepened my understanding of the condition but also highlighted the profound impact it can have on every aspect of one's life. IBS, with its complex interplay of symptoms, stands apart from other gastrointestinal disorders in both its prevalence and its pervasive influence on those it affects.

The journey to managing IBS effectively is fraught with challenges, from the initial uncertainty surrounding its symptoms to the ongoing struggle to find relief. It is a journey that demands not only medical intervention but also a profound personal understanding and adaptation. The cornerstone of this journey is an accurate diagnosis. The importance of distinguishing IBS from other conditions with similar symptoms—such as celiac disease, inflammatory bowel disease, and various food intolerances—cannot be overstated.

This diagnostic process, guided by the Rome IV criteria, is more than a clinical exercise; it's a critical step in crafting a management plan that addresses each individual's unique manifestations of the syndrome. The complexity of IBS, with its variable symptoms and triggers, requires a nuanced approach to management—an approach that is both evidence-based and personalized.

It is from this understanding and a desire to empower those living with IBS that the "IBS Management Blueprint" was conceived. This book is not merely a collection of medical advice but a comprehensive guide aimed at demystifying IBS and providing practical, actionable strategies for managing the condition. The goal is to arm you with the knowledge and tools necessary to navigate the complexities of IBS, enabling you to take control of your symptoms and, by extension, your life. This journey is about more than finding temporary relief; it's about establishing a new normal— a life where IBS is a manageable part of your story, not the defining element.

Navigating your IBS journey is an inherently personal process. It requires a keen awareness of your body's reactions, an understanding of potential triggers, and the flexibility to adapt management strategies as your life and symptoms evolve. This book aims to guide you through this process, offering insights into everything from diet and stress management to medical treatments and alternative therapies. It's about fostering a partnership between you and your healthcare providers, ensuring that your management plan is as dynamic and multifaceted as IBS itself.

This endeavor to write "IBS Management Blueprint" was fueled by the stories and struggles of my patients—their resilience in the face of discomfort, their determination to find solutions, and their courage to make the necessary changes to improve their quality of life. I hope that this book serves as a beacon of hope and a source of strength for you on your IBS journey. Herein lies a pathway to managing symptoms and a roadmap to a life defined not by IBS but by wellness, fulfillment, and joy.

In embarking on this journey together through the pages of this book, I aim to bridge the gap between patient and physician, to translate the complexities of medical science into practical, everyday strategies that can bring relief and empowerment. Your journey with IBS is unique and deserves a personalized approach that honors your individual experiences, challenges, and goals. "IBS Management Blueprint" is more than a guide; it's a companion on your journey to a better quality of life, offering evidence-based advice, compassionate understanding, and, most importantly, hope for the future. Welcome to the first step on this transformative journey.

CHAPTER ONE: UNDERSTANDING IBS

In this chapter, we delve into the complex world of Irritable Bowel Syndrome (IBS), a condition that mystifies many. We'll explore the underlying science that explains why IBS occurs, distinguish between its various types and their specific symptoms, identify common triggers that can provoke flare-ups, and acknowledge the significant psychological impact it has on sufferers. Understanding IBS is the first step toward effective management, empowering you with the knowledge to navigate your symptoms with confidence and clarity.

The Science Behind IBS

Irritable Bowel Syndrome (IBS) is a complex, multifaceted condition that remains one of the most common gastrointestinal disorders encountered in clinical practice. At its core, IBS is characterized by a combination of symptoms including abdominal pain, bloating, and altered bowel habits, such as constipation and diarrhea, which do not have an identifiable organic cause. The pathophysiology of IBS, or the processes by which the disease develops and affects the body, is intricate and involves several key factors, including the gut-brain axis, low-grade inflammation, and alterations in the gut microbiota.

The gut-brain axis refers to the bidirectional communication network that links the enteric nervous system of the gastrointestinal tract with the central nervous system. This axis plays a pivotal role in maintaining gastrointestinal homeostasis and is thought to be significantly disrupted in individuals with IBS. Research has shown that this disruption can lead to changes in gut motility, sensitivity, and secretion, all of which can contribute to the hallmark symptoms of IBS. Stress, a common trigger for IBS symptoms, can exacerbate these disruptions, highlighting the importance of the gut-brain interaction in the manifestation of the syndrome.

In addition to abnormalities in the gut-brain axis, emerging evidence suggests that low-grade inflammation may also contribute to the pathogenesis of IBS. While IBS is not traditionally considered an inflammatory condition like inflammatory bowel disease (IBD), subtle inflammatory changes have been observed in some patients. These may include increased numbers of immune cells in the gut lining and altered levels of cytokines, which are signaling molecules that help regulate the immune response. This low-grade inflammation could sensitize nerve endings in the gut, leading to increased pain perception and altered gut motility, further contributing to the symptoms experienced by patients.

Alterations in the gut microbiota, the complex community of microorganisms residing in the gastrointestinal tract, have also been implicated in IBS. Studies have found differences in the composition of the gut microbiota between individuals with IBS and healthy controls, suggesting that dysbiosis, or an imbalance in these microbial populations, may play a role in symptom development. This dysbiosis can affect the gut's ability to function properly, potentially leading to increased gut permeability (sometimes referred to as "leaky gut"), changes in the production of gut hormones, and alterations in the fermentation of dietary fibers, all of which can influence IBS symptoms.

The interaction between these factors—gut-brain axis dysregulation, low-grade inflammation, and gut microbiota alterations—creates a complex network of pathophysiological processes that contribute to the development and persistence of IBS symptoms. Understanding these underlying mechanisms is crucial for developing targeted therapeutic strategies and managing IBS more effectively. As research continues to unravel the intricacies of IBS, it is hoped that this will lead to more personalized and effective treatments for those affected by this challenging syndrome.

Types of IBS and Their Symptoms

Irritable Bowel Syndrome (IBS) is a complex, multifaceted condition that significantly impacts the lives of those it affects. To understand IBS fully, it is crucial to recognize that it manifests in several subtypes, each defined by the predominant bowel habit of the individual. This classification into subtypes not only aids in the diagnosis and understanding of IBS but also in tailoring treatment approaches to address the specific challenges each subtype presents.

IBS is primarily divided into four subtypes: IBS with predominant constipation (IBS-C), IBS with predominant diarrhea (IBS-D), IBS with mixed bowel habits (IBS-M), and IBS unclassified (IBS-U). Each of these subtypes has a distinct set of symptoms, reflecting the diverse ways in which IBS can affect the gastrointestinal system.

IBS-C is characterized by chronic constipation, where individuals experience infrequent bowel movements, hard or lumpy stools, and often a sensation of incomplete evacuation. This subtype can lead to significant discomfort, abdominal pain, and bloating, with constipation contributing to a feeling of fullness and discomfort in the abdomen. The exact causes of IBS-C include abnormalities in gut motility, increased sensitivity to gas, and alterations in the gut microbiota, which can lead to the slower movement of stool through the colon.

Conversely, IBS-D is marked by frequent, loose, or watery stools and an urgent need to have a bowel movement. Individuals with IBS-D may experience sudden bouts of diarrhea, often accompanied by abdominal pain and cramping. The challenges of managing IBS-D include dealing with the unpredictability of symptoms and the anxiety that can arise from the need to locate restrooms urgently.

The pathophysiology of IBS-D involves increased gut motility, heightened visceral sensitivity, and changes in the intestinal flora, which can lead to rapid transit of stool and increased fluid secretion.

IBS-M, or mixed IBS, presents as a combination of both constipation and diarrhea. Individuals with IBS-M experience alternating patterns of bowel habits, which can make the condition particularly challenging to manage. The variability in symptoms requires a flexible and nuanced approach to treatment, as individuals may experience shifts in the predominant symptom over time. The underlying mechanisms of IBS-M involve fluctuations in gut motility and sensitivity, as well as imbalances in the gut microbiome, contributing to alternating bowel habits.

IBS-U, or unclassified IBS, is designated for individuals whose symptoms do not consistently align with the other three subtypes. This category acknowledges the variability and complexity of IBS, where symptoms may fluctuate or not fit neatly into the categories of constipation or diarrhea dominance. Managing IBS-U requires a personalized approach, focusing on symptom relief and improving the individual's quality of life.

Understanding the specific challenges each IBS subtype presents is crucial for effective management. For IBS-C, treatment may focus on dietary adjustments, such as increasing fiber intake, and medications to enhance bowel movements. For IBS-D, dietary changes to avoid trigger foods, along with medications to reduce diarrhea and manage pain, are common approaches. IBS-M treatment strategies may shift depending on the current predominant symptom, requiring a dynamic and adaptable approach. For IBS-U, treatment is highly individualized, aiming to address the most bothersome symptoms as they arise.

In conclusion, the classification of IBS into subtypes based on predominant bowel habits is essential for understanding the diverse presentations of this syndrome. Each subtype presents unique challenges, necessitating tailored treatment strategies to manage symptoms effectively and improve the quality of life for those affected by IBS.

Common Triggers of IBS Flare-Ups

Navigating the complexities of Irritable Bowel Syndrome (IBS) demands a nuanced understanding of the myriad triggers that can precipitate symptoms. For those afflicted, IBS is not merely a condition but a daily challenge influenced by an array of factors, from the foods consumed to the stressors encountered. A deeper exploration into these triggers, coupled with strategies for identification and management, is essential for crafting a life less encumbered by the unpredictable manifestations of IBS.

Dietary Triggers

The diet of an individual with IBS can significantly influence their symptoms. Beyond the well-known high-FODMAP foods, a variety of other dietary elements have been identified as potential triggers:

- **Complex Carbohydrates**: While certain carbohydrates can exacerbate symptoms, understanding the nuances between different types (e.g., soluble vs. insoluble fiber) is crucial. Soluble fiber can help manage IBS symptoms, whereas insoluble fiber might worsen them in some cases.

- **Fatty Foods**: Foods high in fat can stimulate intense contractions of the colon, leading to diarrhea or discomfort for some individuals with IBS.

- **Fructose**: A sugar found in fruits, honey, and high-fructose corn syrup, fructose can be difficult for people with IBS to absorb fully, leading to gas, bloating, and diarrhea.

- **Spicy Foods**: Capsaicin, present in spicy foods, can irritate the gut lining and exacerbate pain and diarrhea.

Engaging in an elimination diet under the guidance of a healthcare professional or dietitian can help systematically identify food sensitivities. This process involves the careful reintroduction of eliminated foods, one at a time, to observe potential symptom flare-ups. Keeping a comprehensive food and symptom diary, detailing not only what was eaten but also the context and stress levels at the time, can offer insights into specific dietary triggers and their effects on IBS symptoms.

Stress and Emotional Factors

The connection between the gut and the brain is a pivotal aspect of IBS, with stress and emotional health playing significant roles in symptom fluctuation. Psychological stressors can trigger the release of neurotransmitters and hormones that affect gut function, leading to symptom exacerbation. Techniques such as progressive muscle relaxation, biofeedback, and regular engagement in hobbies or activities that foster relaxation can be beneficial. Additionally, psychotherapy, especially cognitive-behavioral therapy, has shown promise in helping individuals with IBS manage stress and develop coping mechanisms.

Hormonal Changes

The interplay between hormones and IBS, particularly in women, suggests a notable sensitivity of the gut to hormonal changes. Progesterone and estrogen, which fluctuate throughout the menstrual cycle, can impact gut motility and sensitivity. For some, symptoms may intensify during menstruation or ovulation. Understanding these patterns can aid in anticipating and mitigating symptom severity through lifestyle adjustments or medication.

Medications and Antibiotics

Medications, while often necessary for other conditions, can inadvertently worsen IBS symptoms. Antibiotics, for instance, can disrupt the delicate balance of the gut microbiome, leading to an overgrowth of harmful bacteria or a reduction in beneficial bacteria, which can trigger or exacerbate symptoms. Proton pump inhibitors (PPIs), used to treat acid reflux, have also been associated with changes in gut flora. Discussing the potential side effects of new medications with a healthcare provider and exploring alternatives or probiotic supplementation can be prudent steps.

Lifestyle and Environmental Triggers

Lifestyle factors, including physical inactivity and insufficient sleep, play critical roles in the management of IBS symptoms. Regular, moderate exercise can improve overall gut function and reduce stress, while a consistent sleep schedule supports the regulation of gut motility. Environmental changes, such as traveling or alterations in daily routine, can disrupt the regularity of bowel habits, underscoring the importance of maintaining routine as much as possible.

Identifying and Managing Personal Triggers

The path to identifying personal IBS triggers is highly individualized and requires a methodical approach. Beyond elimination diets and symptom diaries, engaging with healthcare professionals for targeted tests (e.g., lactose intolerance tests, and fructose malabsorption tests) can provide additional clarity. Support from dietitians, therapists, and IBS support groups can also offer resources and strategies for managing life with IBS.

In crafting a management plan for IBS, the goal is not merely to mitigate symptoms but to enhance the individual's quality of life. Through a comprehensive understanding of the triggers and a personalized approach to diet, stress management, and lifestyle adjustments, individuals with IBS can navigate their condition with greater confidence and control.

The Psychological Impact of IBS

The psychological impact of Irritable Bowel Syndrome (IBS) is profound and multifaceted, reflecting a complex interplay between mental health and physical symptoms. This bidirectional relationship underscores how IBS can not only stem from or exacerbate psychological stressors such as anxiety, depression, and stress but also how these mental health challenges can, in turn, worsen the physical manifestations of IBS. Understanding this intricate connection is crucial for developing effective strategies to manage both the physical and psychological aspects of the syndrome.

The Bidirectional Relationship between IBS and Mental Health

IBS's impact on an individual's life extends far beyond the physical discomfort of its symptoms. The unpredictability of the condition, coupled with the often debilitating nature of its flare-ups, can lead to significant psychological distress. Individuals with IBS frequently report higher levels of anxiety and stress, driven by the constant concern over when and where symptoms may arise. This state of heightened vigilance can exacerbate IBS symptoms, demonstrating the direct impact of psychological factors on the condition.

Depression is another common companion of IBS, with the chronic nature of the syndrome fostering feelings of despair and isolation. The limitations that IBS places on social and professional life can lead to a withdrawal from activities once enjoyed, further deepening the sense of isolation and contributing to depressive symptoms. The social stigma associated with gastrointestinal symptoms can exacerbate this isolation, making individuals reluctant to seek help or share their experiences.

The gut-brain axis plays a pivotal role in this relationship, mediating the communication between the central nervous system and the enteric nervous system. Stress and emotional disturbances can alter gut motility and sensitivity through this axis, leading to an exacerbation of IBS symptoms. This underscores the importance of interventions that target both psychological and physical aspects of the syndrome.

Strategies for Managing the Psychological Impact of IBS

To effectively manage IBS, it is crucial to adopt strategies that address the psychological impact of the condition alongside the physical symptoms.

Cognitive-Behavioral Therapy (CBT)

CBT stands out as a cornerstone in managing the psychological aspects of IBS. By addressing negative thought patterns and behaviors, CBT can significantly reduce stress, anxiety, and depression levels, which in turn can alleviate IBS symptoms. Techniques such as cognitive restructuring help individuals challenge and change maladaptive beliefs about their condition, while behavioral experiments encourage them to gradually face situations they have been avoiding due to fear of triggering symptoms.

Mindfulness-Based Stress Reduction (MBSR)

MBSR programs, which include mindfulness meditation, body awareness, and yoga, can help individuals develop a nonjudgmental awareness of the present moment. This approach can reduce the stress response and its impact on IBS symptoms. Regular mindfulness practice has been shown to decrease the severity of IBS symptoms, improve quality of life, and reduce anxiety and depression.

Regular Physical Activity

Engaging in regular, moderate exercise not only improves physical health but also acts as a powerful stress reliever. Exercise promotes the release of endorphins, which are natural mood elevators, helping to counteract anxiety and depression. Activities should be chosen based on personal preference and tolerance, to integrate exercise as a regular, enjoyable part of the individual's routine.

Building Support Networks

Finding support through groups or communities of individuals facing similar challenges can provide emotional comfort and practical advice for managing IBS. These networks can reduce feelings of isolation and offer a platform for sharing experiences and coping strategies. Psychoeducational resources, including books, workshops, and reputable online content, can further empower individuals by enhancing their understanding of IBS and its management.

Integrative Approaches

Integrating dietary management with psychological interventions can offer comprehensive relief from IBS symptoms. Working with a dietitian to identify and manage food triggers, combined with psychological support to address anxiety and stress, can create a synergistic effect, enhancing overall well-being.

In crafting a detailed and holistic approach to managing IBS, it is crucial to recognize the significant role psychological factors play in the condition. By employing a combination of CBT, MBSR, physical activity, support networks, and integrative approaches, individuals can effectively navigate the challenges of IBS. This multifaceted strategy not only aims to alleviate physical symptoms but also addresses the psychological impact of IBS, paving the way for improved mental health and quality of life.

CHAPTER TWO: DIETARY MANAGEMENT

Diet plays a pivotal role in managing Irritable Bowel Syndrome (IBS), offering a pathway to relief for many sufferers. This chapter explores the critical relationship between diet and IBS, delving into the low-FODMAP diet's principles and its impact on symptoms. We'll guide you through identifying foods that may trigger flare-ups and those that can be safely enjoyed. Additionally, practical advice on constructing an IBS-friendly meal plan will empower you to navigate your dietary choices confidently, aiming for symptom reduction and improved well-being.

The Role of Diet in IBS Management

The nexus between diet and Irritable Bowel Syndrome (IBS) is a subject of paramount importance for those afflicted by this condition. The intricate relationship underscores not just the influence of dietary choices on the manifestation of IBS symptoms but also illuminates the path toward symptom management through careful dietary adjustments. This deep dive into the role of diet in IBS management explores the multifaceted nature of trigger foods, the physiological mechanisms by which they exacerbate symptoms, and the strategic approach to dietary modification for symptom alleviation.

Deciphering Trigger Foods in IBS

Trigger foods are essentially certain types or categories of food that can provoke or amplify the symptoms associated with IBS. These symptoms range from abdominal discomfort, bloating, and gas to more disruptive manifestations like diarrhea and constipation. The specificity of trigger foods can greatly vary across individuals, which underscores the highly personalized nature of dietary management in IBS. Among the broad spectrum of potential triggers, some of the most commonly implicated include foods rich in FODMAPs, lactose-containing dairy products, foods high in fat, caffeine, alcohol, spicy foods, and artificial sweeteners like sorbitol.

Physiological Mechanisms Behind Trigger Foods

The adverse effects of trigger foods on IBS symptoms can be attributed to several key physiological mechanisms:

- **Fermentation and Gas Production**: High-FODMAP foods are notorious for their poor absorption in the small intestine. When these foods transit to the large intestine, they undergo fermentation by resident gut bacteria, resulting in the production of gas. This process can lead to uncomfortable symptoms such as bloating, abdominal distension, and pain due to the accumulation of gas.

- **Osmotic Effects**: The osmotic action of certain foods, particularly those high in FODMAPs, draws water into the intestine, potentially leading to diarrhea by increasing intestinal fluid volume and altering bowel habits.

- **Influence on Gut Motility**: The motility of the gastrointestinal tract can be significantly affected by dietary choices. Fatty and rich foods may decelerate gut motility, contributing to constipation. Conversely, stimulants like caffeine and certain spicy foods can accelerate gut motility, leading to diarrhea.

- **Heightened Visceral Sensitivity**: Many individuals with IBS exhibit an increased visceral sensitivity, making the gut more reactive to the stretching and distension caused by the normal digestive processes. This heightened sensitivity can transform otherwise normal digestive events into painful experiences.

Strategic Dietary Management in IBS

Addressing IBS symptoms through dietary management involves a nuanced approach that begins with the identification and subsequent elimination of potential trigger foods. This is often achieved through structured elimination diets, such as the low-FODMAP diet, which systematically removes foods known to cause symptoms before gradually reintroducing them to identify specific triggers. This phase of reintroduction is critical for determining individual sensitivities and developing a tailored diet that minimizes symptom occurrence.

Beyond the elimination of trigger foods, ensuring a nutritionally balanced diet that promotes gut health is essential. Incorporating a diverse range of well-tolerated foods, ensuring adequate fiber intake for those who can tolerate it, and maintaining a diet low in FODMAPs are foundational steps. Additionally, the inclusion of probiotic-rich foods and those with anti-inflammatory properties can support a healthy gut microbiome, potentially mitigating the severity of IBS symptoms.

Proper dietary management also entails the adoption of healthy eating habits. Eating meals regularly and maintaining a balanced diet can assist in regulating bowel function. Mindful eating practices, such as eating slowly and chewing food thoroughly, can aid in digestion and reduce the likelihood of symptom flare-ups.

In crafting a comprehensive dietary strategy for IBS management, it is crucial to work closely with healthcare professionals, including dietitians specializing in gastrointestinal disorders. This collaboration ensures the development of a personalized dietary plan that not only addresses the avoidance of trigger foods but also secures nutritional adequacy and promotes overall digestive health.

In essence, the role of diet in managing IBS extends beyond mere symptom management to encompass a broader strategy aimed at enhancing the quality of life for those affected. Through a detailed understanding of trigger foods, their physiological impacts, and a strategic approach to diet modification, individuals with IBS can achieve meaningful relief from their symptoms and navigate the condition with greater confidence and control.

FODMAPs and IBS: What You Need to Know

The low FODMAP diet represents a significant advancement in the dietary management of Irritable Bowel Syndrome (IBS), offering a scientifically backed approach to reducing gastrointestinal discomfort associated with this condition. At its core, the diet targets specific types of carbohydrates known to trigger symptoms in sensitive individuals, providing a structured framework for identifying personal dietary triggers and formulating a sustainable, symptom-minimizing eating plan. Delving into the scientific underpinnings, implementation strategies, and inherent limitations of the low FODMAP diet reveals its potential as a transformative tool for individuals grappling with IBS.

The Science Behind the Low FODMAP Diet

The foundation of the low FODMAP diet rests on the principle that certain carbohydrates, due to their structure and digestion process, can exacerbate IBS symptoms. These carbohydrates are categorized as FODMAPs — Fermentable Oligosaccharides, Disaccharides, Monosaccharides, and Polyols. These compounds are poorly absorbed in the small intestine, and when they reach the colon, they become fermented by gut bacteria, producing gas as a byproduct. This gas can cause bloating, pain, and altered bowel habits. Additionally, FODMAPs can draw water into the intestine, leading to diarrhea in some individuals. By reducing the intake of these fermentable carbohydrates, the low FODMAP diet aims to decrease the volume of readily fermentable substrates in the gut, thereby alleviating the symptoms of IBS.

Implementing the Low FODMAP Diet: A Structured Approach

Phase 1: Elimination

The implementation of the low FODMAP diet begins with an elimination phase, typically lasting 4 to 6 weeks, during which all high-FODMAP foods are removed from the diet. This phase demands meticulous attention to food labels and ingredient lists, as FODMAPs are prevalent in a wide array of foods, from certain fruits and vegetables to dairy products, grains, and processed foods. The objective during this period is to achieve a baseline reduction in symptoms, setting the stage for the careful reintroduction of foods in the subsequent phase.

Phase 2: Reintroduction

Following the elimination phase, the reintroduction phase involves systematically reintroducing high-FODMAP foods back into the diet, one group at a time. This process allows individuals to precisely identify which foods or categories of FODMAPs trigger their symptoms. Each food is introduced in small amounts, gradually increasing over several days, with careful monitoring of symptoms. This phase is crucial for determining personal tolerance levels and understanding the specific dietary triggers that exacerbate IBS symptoms.

Phase 3: Personalization

Armed with the knowledge gained during the reintroduction phase, individuals can then personalize their diet in the long-term maintenance phase. This involves incorporating a variety of low-FODMAP foods and reintroducing tolerable high-FODMAP foods in moderation. The goal is to maintain a balanced and nutritionally complete diet that minimizes IBS symptoms while avoiding unnecessary restrictions. Regular reevaluation and adjustment of the diet may be necessary, as tolerance to certain FODMAPs can change over time.

Limitations of the Low FODMAP Diet

Despite its efficacy for many individuals with IBS, the low FODMAP diet is not without its challenges. The diet can be complex and restrictive, particularly in its initial phases, requiring significant dietary adjustments and vigilance. The potential for nutritional deficiencies is a concern, highlighting the importance of professional guidance from a dietitian experienced in managing the low FODMAP diet. Furthermore, the diet does not address non-dietary triggers of IBS, such as stress and anxiety, underscoring the need for a comprehensive approach to IBS management that may include stress-reduction techniques and other lifestyle modifications.

In essence, the low FODMAP diet offers a promising pathway to improved quality of life for individuals with IBS, through a detailed understanding of how diet influences symptoms. By meticulously implementing and personalizing the diet with professional support, individuals can identify their specific dietary triggers, achieve symptom relief, and work towards a more balanced and enjoyable dietary regimen. However, the journey through the phases of the low FODMAP diet requires patience, commitment, and adaptability, with a focus on long-term dietary and lifestyle adjustments to manage IBS effectively.

Foods to Embrace and Avoid

Navigating the dietary landscape when managing Irritable Bowel Syndrome (IBS) requires a careful and informed approach. The relationship between diet and IBS symptoms is well-documented, necessitating an awareness of which foods may trigger symptoms and which can be safely incorporated into one's diet. Here, we delve deeper into the specifics of foods to avoid and embrace, complemented by detailed advice on label reading and strategic food substitutions to aid those with IBS in making informed dietary choices.

List of Foods to Avoid

The avoidance of certain foods is crucial in managing IBS symptoms due to their potential to trigger discomfort and exacerbate conditions. This list provides a more exhaustive look at foods known to cause issues:

High-FODMAP Foods: Fermentable carbohydrates that can exacerbate IBS symptoms due to poor absorption in the small intestine, leading to fermentation in the gut. Detailed examples include:

- **Oligosaccharides**: Common sources are wheat, rye, various legumes, garlic, and onions. These are found in many breads, cereals, and snacks, contributing to gas and bloating.

- **Disaccharides**: Primarily lactose found in dairy products like milk, soft cheeses, and yogurts, which can cause diarrhea, gas, and bloating in lactose-intolerant individuals.

- **Monosaccharides**: Foods high in fructose, such as apples, mangoes, pears, and products containing high-fructose corn syrup, can lead to diarrhea and abdominal pain.

- **Polyols**: Sugar alcohols like sorbitol, mannitol, and xylitol, present in sugar-free gums, candies, and some fruits like avocados and stone fruits, can cause diarrhea.

Dairy Products: Beyond lactose, the fat content in dairy can also be problematic, stimulating the gut and leading to symptoms. Opting for lactose-free or low-fat options can be beneficial.

Gluten-Containing Foods: For some, gluten can exacerbate IBS symptoms. Avoiding wheat, barley, and rye and choosing gluten-free options can help.

Fatty and Fried Foods: Foods high in fat can accelerate intestinal contractions, leading to diarrhea or discomfort. Lean meats and baked or grilled preparations are preferable.

Caffeinated Beverages: Coffee, tea, and certain sodas can irritate the gastrointestinal tract, increasing motility and exacerbating symptoms like diarrhea.

Alcoholic Beverages: Alcohol can irritate the gut lining and affect gut motility, worsening IBS symptoms. Moderation or avoidance is recommended.

Spicy Foods: The capsaicin in spicy foods can irritate the gastrointestinal tract, leading to discomfort and exacerbation of symptoms.

Foods Generally Considered Safe

Incorporating safe foods into the diet can help maintain nutritional balance while managing IBS symptoms. This expanded list includes:

- **Low-FODMAP Fruits and Vegetables**: Kiwi, oranges, strawberries, bell peppers, carrots, and potatoes offer nutritional benefits without the risk of triggering symptoms.

- **Lean Proteins**: Incorporate a wider variety of lean meats, including pork loin and lean cuts of beef, alongside poultry, fish, and plant-based proteins like tempeh.

- **Whole Grains and Starches**: Look for gluten-free options such as buckwheat, millet, and amaranth, which provide fiber and nutrients without triggering symptoms.

- **Nuts and Seeds**: Almonds (in small quantities), macadamia nuts, pumpkin seeds, and chia seeds can be good low-FODMAP options.

- **Dairy Alternatives**: In addition to lactose-free and plant-based kinds of milk, consider kefir and Greek yogurt, which may be easier to digest due to their probiotic content.

Label Reading and Food Substitutions

Label Reading

- **Identify Hidden FODMAPs**: Look for ingredients like fructans, galacto-oligosaccharides (GOS), and polyols in processed foods. These can be hidden in natural flavorings, condiments, and sauces.

- **Check for Additives**: Emulsifiers, preservatives, and artificial colorings can irritate the gut. Ingredients like carrageenan and xanthan gum, often found in dairy alternatives and gluten-free products, may cause issues for some.

- **Sugar Alcohols**: Common in sugar-free products, these can be identified by names ending in "-ol," such as sorbitol, mannitol, and xylitol.

Food Substitutions

- **Fruit and Vegetable Swaps**: Replace high-FODMAP fruits and vegetables with their low-FODMAP counterparts, ensuring variety and nutritional adequacy. Use spinach instead of cauliflower and raspberries instead of cherries, for instance.

- **Protein Choices**: When substituting proteins, opt for grilled or baked preparations over fried to reduce fat content, which can trigger symptoms.

- **Dairy and Grain Alternatives**: Choose lactose-free dairy or fortified plant-based alternatives to ensure calcium and vitamin D intake. When selecting gluten-free grains, opt for those enriched or fortified with B vitamins and iron to compensate for what might be missing from wheat-based products.

Adopting these detailed dietary guidelines involves a commitment to understanding and adjusting one's diet in response to IBS symptoms. It requires vigilance in identifying trigger foods, a willingness to explore safe alternatives, and an ongoing dialogue with healthcare providers to ensure nutritional needs are met. Through careful planning and informed choices, individuals with IBS can achieve a balance between enjoying a varied, nutritious diet and managing their symptoms effectively.

Creating an IBS-Friendly Meal Plan

Creating an IBS-friendly meal plan is a cornerstone of managing Irritable Bowel Syndrome (IBS), tailored to the individual's specific type of IBS (IBS-D, IBS-C, IBS-M, or IBS-U) and their unique response to various foods. This comprehensive approach aims not only to minimize symptoms but also to ensure a nutritionally complete diet. Here, we talk about crafting a personalized meal plan, integrating detailed sample meal plans for different IBS types, providing nuanced tips for dining out, and offering strategies for adapting the meal plan based on symptom response.

Step 1: Identifying Your IBS Type and Trigger Foods

The journey begins with a clear understanding of your IBS subtype. This knowledge serves as the foundation for identifying foods that may trigger your symptoms. An elimination diet, particularly focusing on high-FODMAP foods, is a structured way to identify these triggers. Over a period of 4-6 weeks, eliminate foods high in FODMAPs, then gradually reintroduce them into your diet one at a time, monitoring your body's reaction to pinpoint specific sensitivities.

Step 2: Crafting a Balanced Meal Plan

A balanced, IBS-friendly meal plan incorporates a wide range of foods across all major food groups, customized to avoid identified triggers. Here are sample meal plans for IBS-C (constipation-predominant), IBS-D (diarrhea predominant), and IBS-M (mixed symptoms), each designed to cater to the specific needs of these IBS types. These plans incorporate a variety of foods from all food groups, ensuring a balanced diet while avoiding common triggers.

IBS-C Sample Meal Plans

Meal Plan 1

- **Breakfast**: Start your day with a smoothie made from spinach, a ripe banana for sweetness, and almond milk for a dairy-free base. Add a tablespoon of ground flaxseed for additional fiber to aid digestion.

- **Lunch**: Prepare a nourishing brown rice bowl featuring baked tofu for protein, along with carrots and cucumbers for crunch. Dress with a ginger-tamari sauce that combines the gut-friendly benefits of ginger with the savory depth of tamari.

- **Dinner**: Enjoy a comforting meal of roasted chicken served with baked sweet potatoes, rich in soluble fiber, and a side of steamed broccoli to provide both fiber and nutrients without excessive gas.

- **Snacks**: Opt for orange slices for a vitamin C boost or a small serving of raspberries for their fiber content.

Meal Plan 2:

- **Breakfast**: Overnight oats made with lactose-free milk ensure a gentle start, topped with sliced strawberries for flavor and pumpkin seeds for added fiber and healthy fats.

- **Lunch**: A refreshing lentil salad with diced tomatoes and bell peppers offers a fiber-rich meal, dressed with lemon-olive oil for a simple, IBS-friendly flavoring.

- **Dinner**: Grilled salmon, a great source of omega-3 fatty acids, is paired with quinoa and roasted carrots, combining protein, fiber, and nutrients in a digestible form.

- **Snacks**: Enjoy a handful of grapes for hydration or lactose-free yogurt to support gut health.

Meal Plan 3

- **Breakfast**: Chia pudding made with coconut milk provides a fiber-rich start, topped with kiwi, which is low in FODMAPs and high in vitamin C.

- **Lunch**: A turkey and spinach wrap using a gluten-free tortilla offer a satisfying, low-FODMAP lunch option. Add mustard for flavor and slices of cucumber for freshness.

- **Dinner**: Beef stir-fry with bok choy, bell peppers, and ginger over brown rice delivers a balanced meal with a mix of protein, fiber, and antioxidants.

- **Snacks**: Carrot sticks paired with a tablespoon of peanut butter provide a crunchy, nutritious snack option.

IBS-D Sample Meal Plans

Meal Plan 1

- **Breakfast**: Begin with scrambled eggs and gluten-free toast, accompanied by a side of lactose-free yogurt to introduce probiotics without dairy discomfort.

- **Lunch**: Baked chicken breast with mashed potatoes made with lactose-free milk and a side of sautéed spinach offers a comforting, easy-to-digest meal.

- **Dinner**: Grilled tilapia with a side of rice and steamed green beans provides lean protein and simple carbs for an easy-on-the-stomach evening meal.

- **Snacks**: Choose a banana for a soluble fiber source or a rice cake topped with a thin layer of almond butter for a satisfying snack.

Meal Plan 2

- **Breakfast**: Gluten-free oatmeal made with water and topped with blueberries for antioxidants without high FODMAPs.

- **Lunch**: A quinoa salad with grilled shrimp, cucumber, and a simple olive oil and lemon juice dressing combines protein with low-FODMAP veggies.

- **Dinner**: Turkey meatballs baked and served with gluten-free pasta and a low-FODMAP tomato sauce for a comforting, IBS-friendly version of a classic dish.

- **Snacks**: Sliced cantaloupe for a refreshing snack or a handful of walnuts for omega-3 fatty acids and protein.

Meal Plan 3

- **Breakfast**: Rice porridge with a sprinkle of cinnamon and a drizzle of maple syrup provides a warm, gentle start to the day.

- **Lunch**: A tuna salad made with mayonnaise served on gluten-free bread, with a side salad of lettuce and shredded carrots for an easy-to-digest lunch.

- **Dinner**: Stir-fried chicken with zucchini, carrots, and ginger served over jasmine rice combines lean protein with low-FODMAP vegetables and aromatic ginger to aid digestion.

- **Snacks**: Opt for a hard-boiled egg or a lactose-free cheese stick for protein-rich snack options that are easy on the gut.

IBS-M Sample Meal Plans

Meal Plan 1

- **Breakfast**: Cornflakes with lactose-free milk accompanied by low-FODMAP fruits like grapes to start the day with soluble fiber and minimal risk of triggering symptoms.

- **Lunch**: A grilled chicken Caesar salad with a low-FODMAP dressing and gluten-free croutons provides a balanced midday meal.

- **Dinner**: Baked cod served with roasted potatoes and green beans for a meal rich in protein and low in FODMAPs.

- **Snacks**: Oranges or a slice of cantaloupe offer a refreshing snack option, providing hydration and nutrients without aggravating symptoms.

Meal Plan 2

- **Breakfast**: A frittata made with spinach, tomatoes, and cheddar cheese offers a protein-rich start with the added benefits of vegetables.

- **Lunch**: Sourdough sandwich with turkey, lettuce, and mustard, accompanied by carrot sticks for a satisfying, crunchy addition.

- **Dinner**: Lemon-garlic shrimp served over quinoa with sautéed kale combines the health benefits of seafood with nutrient-dense greens.

- **Snacks**: A handful of peanuts or kiwi provides a quick energy boost and essential nutrients, catering to different phases of IBS-M.

Meal Plan 3

- **Breakfast**: Lactose-free yogurt mixed with chia seeds and topped with strawberries for a fiber-rich, probiotic start to the day.

- **Lunch**: Rice paper rolls filled with tofu, lettuce, carrots, and cucumber, served with a peanut dipping sauce, offer a light yet nutritious meal.

- **Dinner**: Beef and vegetable stew with a mix of potatoes, carrots, and spinach provides a hearty, comforting meal that's easy on the digestive system.

- **Snacks**: Gluten-free crackers paired with cheddar cheese for a savory snack or a small serving of pineapple for a sweet treat.

Tips for Dining Out

- **Research and Plan**: Before dining out, research the menu and identify IBS-friendly options. Consider contacting the restaurant in advance to inquire about accommodating dietary restrictions.

- **Communicate Your Needs**: Clearly communicate your dietary needs to your server, asking for modifications where necessary to avoid trigger foods.

- **Make Safe Choices**: Opt for dishes that are grilled, baked, or steamed, and be cautious of sauces and dressings that may contain high-FODMAP ingredients.

Step 3: Adjusting Your Meal Plan

An IBS-friendly meal plan is dynamic and should be adjusted based on your symptom response. If certain foods consistently trigger symptoms, eliminate them from your diet. Conversely, if you find that you can tolerate a food that is typically problematic for others with IBS, you may include it in moderation. Regularly review and adjust your meal plan as your understanding of your triggers evolves.

Step 4: Continuous Monitoring and Personalization

Maintaining a food and symptom diary is crucial for identifying triggers and adjusting your meal plan. This ongoing log aids in making informed dietary decisions and helps you and your healthcare provider or dietitian tailor your diet to your specific needs. Remember, managing IBS through diet is highly individualized, and a meal plan that works well for one person may not be effective for another.

Creating an IBS-friendly meal plan is an iterative, personalized process that requires patience, observation, and flexibility. By carefully selecting foods that minimize symptoms and monitoring your body's response, you can craft a diet that effectively manages your IBS while ensuring it remains enjoyable and nutritionally balanced. This proactive approach empowers individuals with IBS to lead a healthier, more comfortable life.

CHAPTER THREE: LIFESTYLE MODIFICATIONS

In the journey to manage Irritable Bowel Syndrome (IBS), lifestyle modifications play a crucial role alongside dietary adjustments. This chapter delves into essential practices that can significantly impact symptom management and overall well-being. We'll explore effective stress management techniques, underscore the importance of regular exercise, highlight the role of sleep hygiene in alleviating IBS symptoms, and discuss strategies for balancing work and social life. Together, these components form a holistic approach to living better with IBS, focusing on enhancing quality of life through practical, everyday changes.

Stress Management Techniques

Stress management is an integral component of managing Irritable Bowel Syndrome (IBS), as stress significantly influences the severity and frequency of IBS symptoms. Effective stress management not only aids in alleviating these symptoms but also enhances overall quality of life. Delving deeper into various stress management techniques, this section provides an enriched exploration of mindfulness meditation, deep breathing exercises, and progressive muscle relaxation (PMR), complete with comprehensive step-by-step guides to facilitate practice.

Mindfulness Meditation

Mindfulness meditation encourages an engaged awareness of the present moment, reducing stress by breaking the habitual cycle of preoccupation with past and future concerns. This practice fosters a state of calmness, aiding in the management of IBS symptoms.

Step-by-Step Guide

- **Preparation**: Choose a tranquil environment where interruptions are unlikely. Ensure your phone is silenced and inform others you need undisturbed time.

- **Position**: Sit in a comfortable posture, whether on a cushion with legs crossed or in a chair with feet flat on the ground. Keep your spine straight to promote alertness.

- **Initial Focus**: Gently close your eyes and take several deep breaths. With every breath out, experience a growing sense of relaxation within yourself.

- **Mindful Breathing**: Shift your attention to your breath. Notice the sensation of air flowing in and out of your body, the rise and fall of your abdomen, or the feel of air at your nostrils. This focus anchors you in the present.

- **Handling Distractions**: It's natural for thoughts, emotions, or external sounds to divert your attention. Acknowledge their presence without judgment, then gently redirect your focus back to your breath.

- **Duration and Frequency**: Begin with 5-10 minutes daily. Gradually increase as you become more comfortable, aiming for 20-30 minutes for deeper practice.

Deep Breathing Exercises

Deep breathing, by promoting relaxation of the mind and body, directly impacts the gut-brain axis, potentially easing IBS symptoms.

Step-by-Step Guide

- **Comfortable Setting**: Sit in a relaxed position in a quiet space or lie flat on your back, placing one hand on your chest and the other on your abdomen to monitor your breathing.

- **Inhalation**: Slowly inhale through your nose, concentrating on filling your lungs from the bottom up. Your abdomen should rise significantly, while your chest should move minimally.

- **Breath Holding**: After inhaling, hold your breath for a count of three to five seconds. This pause allows for maximum oxygen absorption.

- **Exhalation**: Exhale slowly and fully through your mouth, engaging your abdominal muscles to ensure complete expulsion of air.

- **Repetition**: Continue this pattern for 5-10 minutes, focusing on the rhythm and feeling of deep breathing. Practice daily or whenever you need stress relief.

Progressive Muscle Relaxation (PMR)

PMR reduces physical tension and psychological stress by systematically tensing and relaxing muscle groups. This technique can be particularly beneficial for IBS sufferers, as stress often manifests as physical tension, exacerbating symptoms.

Step-by-Step Guide

- **Preparatory Relaxation**: Begin by finding a quiet, comfortable space where you can sit or lie down without distractions. Spend a few moments taking deep breaths to initiate a state of relaxation.

- **Sequential Muscle Tensing**: Starting with the muscles in your toes, tightly tense them for about 5-10 seconds. Focus on the sensation of tension.

- **Controlled Relaxation**: Release the tension suddenly, exhaling as you do so. Observe the difference between the feeling of tension and the sensation of relaxation. Enjoy the sensation of the muscles relaxing.

- **Progressive Technique**: Move through the body in a sequence, from the toes upward, including the lower legs, thighs, glutes, abdomen, chest, hands, arms, shoulders, neck, and face. Tense each muscle group firmly (without causing pain), then relax.

- **Integration into Daily Life**: For optimal benefits, practice PMR daily. The technique can be especially helpful before bedtime to alleviate tension and promote restful sleep, or at any time when stress levels rise.

Incorporating these stress management techniques into daily life requires commitment and practice. Over time, mindfulness meditation, deep breathing exercises, and PMR can become valuable tools in your stress reduction arsenal, offering pathways to manage IBS symptoms more effectively. Consistent practice is key to mastering these techniques, leading to enhanced stress resilience, symptom relief, and improved overall well-being.

The Importance of Regular Exercise

The role of regular exercise in managing Irritable Bowel Syndrome (IBS) extends far beyond its general health benefits. Physical activity can play a crucial part in alleviating IBS symptoms, improving quality of life, and enhancing mental well-being. Understanding the types of exercise that may be most beneficial and learning how to incorporate them into a routine without exacerbating symptoms are key components of a holistic approach to IBS management.

Understanding the Impact of Exercise on IBS

Regular physical activity influences IBS management through several key mechanisms:

- **Stress Reduction**: Physical activity serves as a powerful means of alleviating stress. For many with IBS, stress is a significant trigger for symptom flare-ups. Physical activity helps mitigate stress by promoting the release of endorphins, often referred to as the body's natural painkillers and mood elevators. These biochemical changes can help reduce the perception of pain and promote a sense of well-being.

- **Gut Motility Enhancement**: Regular exercise can improve gut motility, which is particularly beneficial for individuals with IBS-C (constipation-predominant IBS). By stimulating the muscles in the gastrointestinal tract, exercise facilitates smoother and more regular bowel movements, addressing one of the primary concerns in constipation-predominant IBS.

- **Immune System Modulation**: Moderate exercise has been shown to have a positive effect on the immune system, which could be beneficial given the suspected links between immune system dysfunction and IBS. Improved immune function may help manage inflammation in the gut, potentially reducing IBS symptoms.

- **Enhancement of Gut Microbiota**: Emerging research suggests that regular physical activity may positively influence the composition of the gut microbiota, promoting a healthier gut environment. This could play a role in alleviating IBS symptoms, as dysbiosis (imbalance in gut bacteria) has been implicated in IBS pathogenesis.

Beneficial Types of Exercise for IBS

When considering exercise for IBS management, the focus should be on moderate, low-impact activities that stimulate the body without causing undue stress to the digestive system. The following are considered most beneficial:

- **Walking**: As a low-impact activity, walking can be easily incorporated into daily routines and adjusted to fit one's fitness level. Regular walks can help reduce stress, improve cardiovascular health, and stimulate bowel movements.

- **Yoga**: Yoga combines physical postures, breathing exercises, and meditation to reduce stress, improve flexibility, and enhance gut health. Certain poses can specifically target abdominal discomfort and aid in digestion.

- **Pilates**: Similar to yoga, Pilates focuses on core strength, flexibility, and mindful movement. It can help in strengthening the muscles around the abdomen and improving bowel function without a high impact on the body.

- **Swimming**: Swimming and water aerobics are gentle on the body and particularly beneficial for those with joint issues or those who prefer a non-weight-bearing exercise. The buoyancy of water reduces strain on the body while providing an effective cardiovascular workout.

- **Cycling**: Stationary or gentle cycling can be a good option for those looking for a cardiovascular workout without the high impact of running or jogging.

Incorporating Exercise into Your Routine

Incorporating exercise into your routine requires thoughtful consideration of your current fitness level, symptom triggers, and preferences:

- **Gradual Introduction**: Start with low-intensity activities and gradually increase intensity and duration as your body adapts. This cautious approach helps prevent symptom flare-ups.

- **Symptom Monitoring**: Keep a diary to note how different types of exercise affect your IBS symptoms. This will help you identify the activities that benefit you the most.

- **Consistency Over Intensity**: Aim for regular, moderate activity rather than sporadic, intense workouts. Consistency in exercising can help your body adjust and manage symptoms more effectively.

- **Hydration and Nutrition**: Pay attention to hydration and nutritional needs, especially around exercise sessions. Staying hydrated is crucial, and choosing easily digestible, IBS-friendly snacks before and after workouts can help maintain energy levels and prevent digestive discomfort.

- **Incorporating Mindfulness and Relaxation**: In addition to physical activity, include practices that focus on relaxation and stress management, such as meditation or deep breathing exercises, as part of your exercise routine.

Regular exercise, when appropriately tailored to the individual's needs and capabilities, can be a powerful component of an effective IBS management strategy. It offers a holistic approach to alleviating symptoms, enhancing physical health, and improving emotional well-being. As always, consult with healthcare professionals before embarking on a new exercise regimen, particularly if you have concerns about how physical activity may interact with your IBS or other health conditions.

Sleep Hygiene for IBS Sufferers

Improving sleep hygiene for individuals suffering from Irritable Bowel Syndrome (IBS) is crucial, as sleep disturbances often exacerbate the condition's symptoms, creating a challenging cycle of discomfort and restlessness. The intricate relationship between sleep quality and IBS underscores the need for targeted strategies to enhance sleep, thereby potentially mitigating IBS symptoms and improving overall well-being. This exploration delves into detailed strategies for optimizing sleep hygiene, focusing on establishing a conducive sleep environment, adhering to a consistent sleep schedule, and making lifestyle adjustments tailored to the unique challenges faced by IBS sufferers.

Understanding the Sleep-IBS Connection

Sleep disturbances, including difficulty falling asleep, staying asleep, or experiencing non-restorative sleep, are common among those with IBS. These disturbances can stem from nighttime IBS symptoms, such as abdominal pain, bloating, or frequent trips to the bathroom. Conversely, poor sleep can amplify the body's stress response, increase sensitivity to pain, and disrupt the gut-brain axis, exacerbating IBS symptoms. Addressing sleep quality is, therefore, a pivotal aspect of managing IBS effectively.

Advanced Strategies for Enhancing Sleep Hygiene

Developing a Consistent Sleep Routine

- **Set Fixed Sleep and Wake Times**: Establishing a regular sleep schedule trains your body's internal clock to expect sleep at a certain time, aiding in quicker sleep onset and more restful nights.

- **Craft a Pre-Sleep Ritual**: Engage in relaxing activities an hour before bed, such as reading, journaling, or gentle yoga, to signal to your body that it's time to wind down. This ritual can help ease the transition between wakefulness and sleep.

Optimizing the Sleep Environment

- **Invest in Quality Bedding**: Ensure your mattress and pillows support your preferred sleeping position and comfort needs. The right bedding can prevent physical discomfort that might disrupt sleep.

- **Control Ambient Conditions**: Keep your bedroom dark, quiet, and cool. Use blackout curtains to block external light, white noise machines to drown out disruptive sounds, and adjust the thermostat to a cooler temperature conducive to sleep.

- **Limit Exposure to Blue Light**: Reduce screen time at least an hour before bedtime, as blue light from devices can inhibit the production of melatonin, the hormone responsible for regulating sleep.

Lifestyle Modifications for Sleep Improvement

- **Dietary Considerations**: Avoid heavy, spicy, or high-fat meals in the evening that might trigger IBS symptoms. Opt for lighter, easily digestible meals to minimize discomfort. Limit caffeine and alcohol intake in the hours leading up to bedtime, as both can disrupt sleep patterns.

- **Evening Fluid Intake**: While hydration is important, moderating fluid intake in the evening can reduce nighttime bathroom visits. Aim to consume most of your daily fluid intake earlier in the day.

- **Physical Activity**: Incorporate regular, moderate exercise into your daily routine to promote better sleep. Exercise can improve mood, decrease stress, and support regular bowel movements, all of which can contribute to better sleep quality. Nevertheless, it's advisable to refrain from engaging in intense exercise sessions shortly before bedtime, as they may prove overly stimulating.

Addressing Nighttime IBS Symptoms

- **Manage Evening IBS Triggers**: If specific foods are known to trigger your IBS symptoms, avoid them in your evening meal. Consider a low-FODMAP snack if needed before bed to prevent hunger without triggering symptoms.
- **Relaxation Techniques**: Practice relaxation techniques such as progressive muscle relaxation or guided imagery to ease both the mind and body, reducing the likelihood of IBS flare-ups due to stress.

Incorporating Mindfulness and Relaxation Exercises

- **Mindfulness Meditation**: Practice mindfulness meditation to enhance your ability to relax and fall asleep. Focus on your breath and allow thoughts to pass without engagement, fostering a state of calm.

- **Progressive Muscle Relaxation (PMR)**: Before bed, systematically tense and relax each muscle group, starting from your toes and moving upwards. This practice has the potential to alleviate physical tension and foster a sense of relaxation.

Creating a restful sleep environment and routine is essential for individuals with IBS, as quality sleep can significantly impact symptom management and overall quality of life. These detailed strategies offer a roadmap for improving sleep hygiene through careful planning, environmental adjustments, and lifestyle modifications. Tailoring these strategies to fit personal preferences and IBS triggers is key to finding what works best for each individual. As improvements in sleep hygiene are made, many find their ability to manage IBS symptoms during the day also improves, highlighting the integral role of sleep in overall health management.

Balancing Work and Social Life

Successfully managing Irritable Bowel Syndrome (IBS) in both professional and social settings requires strategic planning, effective communication, and self-awareness. As individuals navigate the complexities of work responsibilities and social interactions, the unpredictability of IBS symptoms can be a source of anxiety and stress.

However, with detailed planning and proactive management strategies, it's possible to minimize the impact of IBS on daily life. This section delves deeper into the nuances of managing IBS at work and in social situations, offering more detailed advice on communicating needs, navigating social dining and travel, and maintaining a balanced work-life dynamic.

Communicating Needs in Professional Settings

The professional environment requires careful negotiation when managing a condition like IBS:

- **Document Your Needs**: Prepare a written statement outlining your IBS condition, how it may affect your work and specific accommodations that could help you maintain productivity. This documentation can be helpful during discussions with your employer.

- **Schedule a Formal Meeting**: Request a formal meeting with your supervisor or HR representative to discuss your needs. This ensures the conversation is given the attention and privacy it deserves.

- **Provide Educational Resources**: Some employers may not be familiar with IBS. Providing educational resources or information from reputable sources can help them understand the condition and why certain accommodations are necessary.

- **Follow Up**: After your meeting, send a thank-you email summarizing the discussion and agreed-upon accommodations. This provides a written record and shows your appreciation for their understanding and support.

Navigating Social Dining

Social dining poses specific challenges for those with IBS, requiring more nuanced strategies:

- **Identify Safe Foods**: Develop a list of "safe" foods that you know are unlikely to trigger your IBS symptoms. Share this list with friends or colleagues when they're choosing a restaurant or planning a meal.

- **Offer to Pick the Restaurant**: When possible, volunteer to select the restaurant. This allows you to choose a place that you know can accommodate your dietary needs.

- **Consider Dietary Apps**: Use smartphone apps designed to help identify IBS-friendly foods and restaurants. These tools can make dining out less stressful and more enjoyable.

- **Bring Your Food**: For social gatherings at someone's home, consider bringing a dish you know is safe for you to eat. This not only ensures you'll have something you can eat but also introduces others to your dietary considerations in a positive way.

Managing IBS While Traveling

Travel requires forward-thinking and contingency planning:

- **Create an IBS Travel Kit**: Pack a kit that includes medications, over-the-counter remedies, a water bottle, and safe snacks. Also, include a copy of your medical information and a list of your triggers.

- **Research and Reserve**: Before traveling, spend time researching your destination for accommodations, restaurants, and even local health facilities that are familiar with treating IBS. Make reservations at accommodations that offer the amenities you need to manage your condition comfortably.

- **Plan for Transit**: If traveling by plane or long distances by car, plan how you'll manage your IBS symptoms. Choose aisle seats for easier bathroom access and bring along any documentation that might expedite access to facilities.

- **Stay Flexible**: While having a plan is crucial, remaining flexible and adaptive to changing situations is equally important. Know that it's okay to adjust your plans based on how you're feeling.

Strategies for Work-Life Balance

Achieving a balance necessitates acknowledging your limits and communicating them effectively:

- **Educate Your Circle**: Educate close friends and colleagues about IBS, helping them understand your condition and how they can support you during social or work-related activities.

- **Embrace Flexibility in Commitments**: Give yourself permission to decline invitations or leave events early if you're not feeling well. Being upfront about your condition can help manage expectations.

- **Incorporate Relaxation Techniques**: Regularly practice relaxation techniques that specifically address the stress component of IBS, such as guided imagery or autogenic training, to maintain a calm mindset amidst work and social commitments.

Balancing the demands of work and social life with the management of IBS symptoms is a multifaceted challenge that requires open communication, detailed planning, and self-care. By adopting these comprehensive strategies, individuals with IBS can navigate professional and social settings more effectively, ensuring they lead fulfilling lives while managing their condition.

CHAPTER FOUR: MEDICAL AND ALTERNATIVE THERAPIES

In the journey to manage Irritable Bowel Syndrome (IBS), a comprehensive approach encompassing both medical and alternative therapies offers a beacon of hope for those seeking relief. This chapter delves into the array of treatments available, from conventional medications designed to alleviate IBS symptoms to the nurturing role of probiotics in maintaining gut health.

Furthermore, it explores the significant impact of psychological therapies in addressing the mind-gut connection and investigates the potential benefits of alternative treatments such as acupuncture and herbal remedies. Together, these modalities provide a holistic framework for navigating the complexities of IBS management.

Medications Used in IBS Treatment

Managing Irritable Bowel Syndrome (IBS) often involves a multifaceted approach, with medication playing a crucial role for many sufferers. The goal of pharmacological treatment is to alleviate the symptoms of IBS, such as abdominal pain, bloating, constipation, and diarrhea. Various classes of medications are used, each targeting different symptoms and mechanisms within the gut. This section covers the primary categories of medications commonly prescribed for IBS, including their intended effects, potential side effects, and considerations for long-term use.

Antispasmodics

Antispasmodics are medications designed to reduce muscle spasms in the gastrointestinal tract, which can alleviate abdominal pain and cramping associated with IBS. They work by relaxing the smooth muscle of the gut, thereby reducing the intensity and frequency of spasms.

- **Common Examples**: Dicyclomine (Bentyl) and hyoscine (Scopolamine).
- **Intended Effects**: These medications aim to provide relief from the cramping and pain that IBS patients frequently experience.
- **Potential Side Effects**: Antispasmodics can cause dry mouth, dizziness, blurred vision, and constipation. Because they may affect other smooth muscles in the body, they can also lead to urinary retention and a decrease in sweating.
- **Considerations for Use**: Antispasmodics are often used on an as-needed basis, and taken before meals to prevent symptoms. They may not be suitable for long-term use due to their side effects, especially in older patients or those with certain medical conditions.

Laxatives

For IBS sufferers with predominant constipation (IBS-C), laxatives can help to improve bowel movements and alleviate discomfort. Laxatives work by softening the stool, increasing stool volume, or stimulating bowel movements through various mechanisms.

- **Common Examples**: Polyethylene glycol (Miralax), bisacodyl (Dulcolax), and senna (Senokot).
- **Intended Effects**: Laxatives are intended to ease constipation by facilitating more regular and softer bowel movements.
- **Potential Side Effects**: Overuse of stimulant laxatives can lead to dependency and potentially damage the colon. Other side effects may include bloating, gas, and in some cases, diarrhea.
- **Considerations for Use**: It's crucial to use laxatives as directed and to choose the type that's best suited to your needs. Osmotic laxatives are often recommended for IBS-C due to their gentler action on the gut.

Antidiarrheals

For those with diarrhea-predominant IBS (IBS-D), antidiarrheal medications can help to slow bowel movements and increase stool consistency.

- **Common Examples**: Loperamide (Imodium) is the most commonly used antidiarrheal for IBS-D.

- **Intended Effects**: Antidiarrheals work by slowing the movement of fecal matter through the intestines, allowing more water to be absorbed from the stool.

- **Potential Side Effects**: Possible side effects include constipation, abdominal cramping, and dizziness. Long-term use can lead to dependency and decreased effectiveness.

- **Considerations for Use**: Antidiarrheals should be used cautiously, ideally on an as-needed basis to manage acute diarrhea rather than for continuous long-term use.

Antidepressants

Low doses of antidepressants are prescribed for their pain-modulating effects in the gut, rather than for their effect on mood. They can be particularly effective for IBS sufferers whose symptoms include significant pain or for those with coexisting anxiety or depression.

- **Common Examples**: Tricyclic antidepressants (TCAs) like amitriptyline and SSRIs (selective serotonin reuptake inhibitors) such as fluoxetine (Prozac).

- **Intended Effects**: These medications can help modulate pain perception in the gut and improve overall bowel function.

- **Potential Side Effects**: Side effects can vary between drug classes; TCAs may cause drowsiness, dry mouth, and constipation, while SSRIs can lead to insomnia, nausea, and diarrhea.

- **Considerations for Use**: The dose of antidepressants for IBS is typically lower than that used for treating depression. It's important to have regular follow-ups with a healthcare provider to monitor the effectiveness and adjust the dosage as needed.

When considering medications for IBS treatment, it's essential to work closely with a healthcare provider to tailor the approach based on individual symptoms, response to treatment, and potential side effects. Medication can be a valuable tool in managing IBS, but it's often most effective when combined with dietary changes, lifestyle modifications, and other therapies tailored to the individual's needs.

Probiotics and Gut Health

Probiotics, which derive from the Greek words "pro" (meaning "for") and "bios" (meaning "life"), are living microorganisms that, when consumed in adequate quantities, confer health benefits to the host. These beneficial microorganisms, predominantly bacteria and yeast, are widely recognized for their role in supporting various aspects of gut health. Probiotics can be naturally found in fermented foods such as yogurt, kefir, sauerkraut, and kimchi. Additionally, they are available in various dietary supplements, offering a convenient means of supplementation.

Evidence for Using Probiotics in IBS Management

The utilization of probiotics as a therapeutic intervention for managing symptoms associated with Irritable Bowel Syndrome (IBS) has garnered considerable attention within the scientific community. Numerous clinical trials and meta-analyses have investigated the efficacy of probiotics in alleviating the diverse array of symptoms experienced by individuals with IBS, including abdominal pain, bloating, altered bowel habits, and diminished quality of life. While the outcomes of these studies have exhibited variability, with some trials reporting significant improvements and others demonstrating more modest effects, the collective body of evidence underscores the potential of probiotics as a promising adjunctive therapy for IBS management.

Mechanism of Action

The mechanisms underlying the therapeutic effects of probiotics in the context of IBS are multifaceted and not yet fully elucidated. However, several plausible mechanisms have been proposed based on existing research findings. Foremost among these is the modulation of the gut microbiota, wherein probiotics may exert beneficial effects by restoring microbial balance, ameliorating dysbiosis, and enhancing microbial diversity within the gut ecosystem. Furthermore, probiotics have been implicated in modulating immune responses, attenuating gut inflammation, fortifying gut barrier function, and producing bioactive metabolites such as short-chain fatty acids (SCFAs), all of which contribute to the mitigation of IBS symptoms.

Strains That Have Shown Promise

The vast diversity of probiotic strains available necessitates careful consideration when selecting strains for IBS management. While numerous strains have been explored in clinical trials, several strains have demonstrated consistent efficacy and merit particular attention:

- **Lactobacillus plantarum:** This strain has exhibited notable efficacy in reducing abdominal pain and bloating, thereby offering potential relief for individuals with IBS.

- **Bifidobacterium infantis:** Studies have revealed the capacity of B. infantis to ameliorate overall IBS symptoms, particularly in individuals with diarrhea-predominant IBS (IBS-D), highlighting its relevance as a therapeutic option.

- **Lactobacillus acidophilus:** Evidence suggests that L. acidophilus may exert beneficial effects on symptoms such as abdominal discomfort and irregular bowel movements, rendering it a potentially valuable addition to IBS management strategies.

- **Bifidobacterium longum:** This strain has demonstrated promise in alleviating abdominal pain and improving stool consistency, indicating its potential utility in the management of IBS symptoms.

Guidelines for Selecting and Using Probiotics

Given the diversity and complexity of probiotic products available, adherence to specific guidelines is crucial to optimize their efficacy and ensure safety:

- **Strain specificity:** Consideration of the specific strain(s) employed in a probiotic product is essential, as different strains may exhibit varying effects on IBS symptoms. Select strains with documented efficacy and compatibility with individual needs.

- **Formulation considerations:** Probiotics are available in various formulations, including capsules, tablets, powders, and fermented foods. Choose a formulation that aligns with personal preferences and tolerability.

- **Dosage optimization:** Determining the optimal dosage of probiotics necessitates consideration of factors such as strain potency, individual response variability, and the severity of IBS symptoms. Adhere to manufacturer recommendations or seek guidance from healthcare professionals to ascertain appropriate dosing regimens.

- **Quality assurance:** Prioritize probiotic products that undergo rigorous testing for potency, purity, and safety. Look for products that adhere to established quality standards, such as Good Manufacturing Practices (GMP), and consider third-party certifications for added assurance.

- **Duration and consistency:** Recognize that the benefits of probiotic supplementation may require sustained usage over an extended period to manifest fully. Maintain consistency in probiotic intake and monitor symptom responses to gauge efficacy over time.

In summary, probiotics represent a promising adjunctive approach for the management of Irritable Bowel Syndrome (IBS), offering the potential to ameliorate symptoms and enhance overall gut health. While the precise mechanisms underlying their therapeutic effects warrant further elucidation, the existing body of evidence underscores their relevance in IBS management.

By carefully selecting appropriate probiotic strains, adhering to established guidelines for usage, and maintaining consistency in supplementation, individuals with IBS can potentially harness the benefits of probiotics to alleviate symptoms and improve their quality of life. Continued research endeavors aimed at elucidating the intricate interplay between probiotics and gut health in the context of IBS will further enhance our understanding and inform more refined therapeutic strategies in the future.

The Role of Psychological Therapies

The role of psychological therapies in managing Irritable Bowel Syndrome (IBS) is increasingly recognized as a vital component of a comprehensive treatment plan. Psychological interventions, such as cognitive-behavioral therapy (CBT), gut-directed hypnotherapy, and mindfulness-based stress reduction (MBSR), offer promising avenues for alleviating the burden of IBS.

These therapies address the intricate interplay between the brain and the gut, providing strategies to manage the psychological stressors that can exacerbate IBS symptoms. This section delves into the nuances of these therapies, exploring their mechanisms, effectiveness, and practical application in the context of IBS management.

Cognitive-Behavioral Therapy (CBT)

CBT is a well-established psychological intervention that targets the cognitive and behavioral aspects of emotional distress, which can, in turn, influence IBS symptoms. It operates on the premise that negative thought patterns and maladaptive behaviors contribute to the persistence of IBS symptoms by amplifying stress and anxiety.

- **Mechanism and Application**: CBT for IBS typically involves identifying and challenging negative thought patterns related to the condition, such as catastrophizing pain or discomfort, and replacing them with more balanced, constructive ways of thinking. Additionally, it incorporates behavioral techniques such as relaxation training and stress management to directly address the physiological responses to stress that can trigger or worsen IBS symptoms.

- **Effectiveness**: Numerous clinical trials have demonstrated the efficacy of CBT in reducing the severity of IBS symptoms, including abdominal pain, bloating, and altered bowel habits. It has also been shown to improve quality of life and psychological well-being. The benefits of CBT can persist long after the completion of therapy, offering a durable strategy for managing IBS.

- **Considerations for Use**: While CBT is highly effective, access to qualified therapists and the time commitment required for therapy sessions can be barriers for some individuals. Online CBT programs have emerged as accessible alternatives, showing promise in delivering comparable benefits to traditional face-to-face therapy.

Gut-Directed Hypnotherapy

Gut-directed hypnotherapy is a specialized form of hypnotherapy that focuses specifically on the gastrointestinal tract, aiming to reduce gut sensitivity and normalize digestive function. This therapy is grounded in the concept of the gut-brain axis, which highlights the bidirectional communication between the central nervous system and the enteric nervous system.

- **Mechanism and Application**: Through a series of guided sessions, a trained hypnotherapist helps the individual enter a state of deep relaxation. In this state, the therapist delivers suggestions aimed at calming the digestive system and reducing sensitivity to pain and discomfort. Techniques may include visualizations of the digestive process working smoothly and suggestions for pain management.

- **Effectiveness**: Clinical research supports the use of gut-directed hypnotherapy in significantly reducing IBS symptoms, including abdominal pain, bloating, and irregular bowel movements. It has been particularly beneficial for individuals who have not responded well to conventional medical treatments, offering an alternative path to symptom relief.

- **Considerations for Use**: Gut-directed hypnotherapy requires sessions with a trained hypnotherapist familiar with IBS and its treatment. The therapy can be time-intensive and may require a financial investment, but many find the improvement in symptoms and quality of life to be well worth the commitment.

Mindfulness-Based Stress Reduction (MBSR)

MBSR is a structured program that teaches mindfulness meditation and yoga to reduce stress and improve emotional regulation. By fostering a non-judgmental awareness of the present moment, MBSR helps individuals with IBS manage the stress and anxiety that can aggravate their symptoms.

- **Mechanism and Application**: The MBSR program typically spans eight weeks and includes group sessions that teach various mindfulness practices, including sitting meditation, body scanning, and gentle yoga. Participants are encouraged to practice these techniques daily to cultivate mindfulness and reduce stress.

- **Effectiveness**: Studies on MBSR have shown promising results in alleviating IBS symptoms, reducing the intensity of pain, and improving bowel regularity. Participants often report enhanced emotional well-being and a greater ability to cope with the stressors that can trigger IBS flare-ups.

- **Considerations for Use**: MBSR programs are widely available and can be accessed through certified instructors in community settings or online. Commitment to regular practice is essential for achieving the full benefits of MBSR.

In conclusion, psychological therapies like CBT, gut-directed hypnotherapy, and MBSR play a critical role in the multidimensional management of IBS. By addressing the psychological underpinnings of the condition, these therapies offer valuable tools for alleviating symptoms, enhancing coping mechanisms, and ultimately improving the overall quality of life for individuals with IBS. Their implementation should be personalized, taking into account the individual's specific symptoms, preferences, and lifestyle, and ideally, be integrated into a broader treatment plan that includes dietary management, physical activity, and medical interventions as necessary.

Exploring Alternative Treatments

In the realm of Irritable Bowel Syndrome (IBS) management, the exploration of alternative treatments such as acupuncture and herbal remedies has gained prominence. These approaches, rooted in centuries-old practices, offer a complementary perspective to conventional medical treatments, focusing on the body's natural healing processes and the holistic management of symptoms. This exploration delves into the intricacies of acupuncture and herbal remedies for IBS treatment, evaluating the scientific evidence, discussing the integration of these treatments into a comprehensive management strategy, addressing safety concerns, and offering guidance on selecting qualified practitioners.

Acupuncture in the Management of IBS

Acupuncture, an ancient component of traditional Chinese medicine, operates on the principle of stimulating specific points on the body to correct imbalances in the flow of Qi (energy) through meridians. In the context of IBS, acupuncture is posited to modulate gut motility, alleviate abdominal pain, and mitigate the stress and psychological distress that often exacerbate IBS symptoms.

- **Scientific Evidence and Mechanisms**: The scientific community has shown increasing interest in understanding the mechanisms by which acupuncture might benefit IBS sufferers. Clinical studies and systematic reviews provide mixed evidence, with some trials highlighting significant improvements in IBS symptoms such as abdominal pain, bloating, and bowel habit regularity, while others suggest minimal differences compared to sham (placebo) acupuncture. Theories suggest acupuncture may modulate the autonomic nervous system, reduce inflammation, and enhance the gut-brain axis's functioning, thereby improving gastrointestinal symptoms and overall well-being.

- **Integrating Acupuncture into IBS Treatment Plans**: Acupuncture can complement dietary interventions, pharmacological treatments, and psychological therapies in a holistic IBS management plan. It is particularly appealing for individuals seeking non-pharmacological options and those with a preference for integrative medicine approaches.

- **Safety and Practitioner Selection**: Generally considered safe when conducted by trained, certified practitioners, acupuncture's adverse effects are rare and typically mild. Ensuring practitioners use sterile, single-use needles is paramount to avoid infection. Certification by recognized acupuncture or traditional Chinese medicine regulatory bodies is a key indicator of a practitioner's qualifications.

Herbal Remedies for IBS Symptom Relief

Herbal medicine offers a diverse array of plant-based treatments for various ailments, with several herbs and formulations showing potential benefits for IBS management.

Evidence and Promising Herbs:

- **Peppermint Oil**: Among the most studied herbal remedies for IBS, peppermint oil capsules (enteric-coated to prevent dissolution in the stomach) have consistently demonstrated efficacy in reducing abdominal pain and bloating, attributed to its antispasmodic effects on the gastrointestinal tract.

- **Iberogast® (STW 5)**: This proprietary blend of nine herbs, including chamomile and milk thistle, has been researched for its effectiveness in managing IBS and functional dyspepsia symptoms, offering improvements in pain, bloating, and motility.

- **Chinese Herbal Formulas**: Customized herbal mixtures prescribed in traditional Chinese medicine, tailored to the individual's symptom pattern and constitution, have shown promise in clinical trials for improving IBS symptoms, although variability in formulas makes standardized evaluation challenging.

Incorporating Herbal Remedies into Comprehensive Care: Herbal treatments can be valuable adjuncts to conventional IBS management strategies. Open communication with healthcare providers is crucial to ensure that herbal remedies complement prescribed treatments without adverse interactions. Monitoring efficacy and adjusting treatments as part of an ongoing care plan is essential for optimal outcomes.

Safety Considerations and Quality Assurance: While natural, herbal remedies are not without risks. Variability in herb quality, potential side effects, and interactions with medications necessitate careful consideration. Sourcing products from reputable suppliers and consulting healthcare professionals knowledgeable in herbal medicine are critical steps for safe use.

Finding Qualified Herbal Practitioners: Consulting with qualified herbalists or integrative medicine practitioners with expertise in gastrointestinal disorders can provide personalized herbal treatment recommendations. Credentials in herbal medicine and professional affiliations with reputable herbal or integrative medicine organizations are indicators of a practitioner's expertise.

In summary, acupuncture and herbal remedies represent valuable components of a multidimensional approach to IBS management, offering potential benefits for symptom relief and enhancing quality of life. The integration of these alternative treatments into broader IBS management plans should be approached judiciously, with attention to scientific evidence, safety considerations, and the guidance of qualified professionals. By doing so, individuals with IBS can explore these complementary therapies as part of a holistic strategy aimed at achieving optimal health and well-being.

CONCLUSION

Living with Irritable Bowel Syndrome (IBS) is undeniably challenging, yet it opens a pathway to understanding and nurturing one's body in ways previously unimagined. This book has traversed the landscape of IBS, from understanding its complexities to navigating the myriad treatment options, and the overarching message is one of hope and empowerment. Embracing a life with IBS requires a shift in perspective, where setbacks become opportunities for learning and growth. The journey towards managing IBS is deeply personal, marked by trials and triumphs that uniquely tailor management strategies to each individual's life. It's a path that demands patience, as finding the right combination of diet, medication, and lifestyle changes can be an exercise in trial and error, yet it is through this process that many find their stride in living more fully, despite their condition.

The encouragement to continue exploring and experimenting with various management techniques cannot be overstated. The realms of medical research and alternative therapies are ever-evolving, offering new insights and treatments that could potentially ease the burden of IBS. Engaging in self-care practices plays a critical role in this journey. Activities that promote relaxation, reduce stress, and bring joy are not just supplementary; they are foundational to improving quality of life. This exploration of self-care extends beyond physical health, encompassing mental and emotional well-being, underscoring the importance of addressing the psychological impacts of living with a chronic condition.

Navigating life with IBS is not a solitary journey. A wealth of resources and communities exists to support those affected by this condition. From healthcare professionals who provide guidance and care, to support groups that offer understanding and camaraderie, the network of support is vast and varied. Educational materials, patient advocacy organizations, and online forums further enrich this landscape, providing information and connection. For those seeking to complement traditional medicine with alternative treatments, qualified practitioners in fields such as acupuncture and herbal medicine can offer additional avenues for relief and healing.

In conclusion, while IBS may pose significant challenges, it also presents opportunities for individuals to become advocates for their health, learn resilience, and discover a depth of strength they may not have known they possessed. The key lies in embracing a proactive approach to management, remaining open to new possibilities, and nurturing a compassionate understanding of oneself. With the right support and a commitment to self-care, living positively with IBS is not only achievable but can also lead to a richer, more informed experience of life.